Dr. Earl Mindell's

What You Should Know About Nutrition for Active Lifestyles

Dr. Earl Mindell's

What You Should Know About Nutrition for Active Lifestyles

Earl L. Mindell, R.Ph., Ph.D.

with Virginia L. Hopkins

Dr. Earl Mindell's What You Should Know About Nutrition for Active Lifestyles is intended solely for informational and educational purposes, and not as medical advice. Please consult a medical or health professional if you have questions about your health.

DR. EARL MINDELL'S WHAT YOU SHOULD KNOW ABOUT NUTRITION FOR ACTIVE LIFESTYLES

Copyright © 1996 by Earl L. Mindell, R.Ph., Ph.D.

All Rights Reserved

No part of this book may be reproduced in any form without the written consent of the publisher.

Printed in the United States of America

Book Margins, Inc.
A BMI Edition

By arrangement with Keats Publishing, Inc.

Contents

Introduction 1

1 Reclaiming Your Energy by
  Balancing Your Hormones 5
2 Getting a Good Night's Sleep 17
3 Supplements for a Strong
  Immune System 29
4 Are Allergies Bringing You Down? 39
5 Boosting Energy and Brain Power
  Naturally 47
6 Beating Depression Naturally 59
7 Working with Your Mind and Body
  to Beat Stress 67
Index 78

Dr. Earl Mindell's

What You Should
Know About
Nutrition for
Active Lifestyles

INTRODUCTION

Staying Healthy with an Active Lifestyle

I like to live my life to its full potential, and to do that I maximize my energy and minimize the impact stress has on my life. I often refer to stress as "crunch times." We all have crunch times, and not always for negative reasons—like the positive experience of my annual whistle stop book tours where I'm in eight cities in ten days. The goal of getting through a book tour with my health intact inspires me to pull out all of my antistress tricks. I'm happy to tell you that they work. I accomplish a tremendous amount in a very short time, working from the wee small hours until late at night, and stay healthy and energetic throughout.

Stress can also come in bad packages. Disease, holidays, anxiety, even moving, can burn you out before you realize it. The problem for many people during crunch times begins when they start to feel overwhelmed by life's demands and don't do anything to remedy it. It's at this point that they start to feel serious stress and suffer the physical and emotional consequences, like inability to sleep, gaining or losing weight, exhaustion, irritability, depression and loss of emotional control. Physical symptoms can range from minor aches and pains to considerable chronic and acute conditions.

Physicians in general practice have reported that at least 75 percent of their patients have problems with an emotional beginning. High blood pressure, colitis, heart disease, even cancer have been attributed in large part to poorly managed, chronic stress.

I'm not saying avoid stress—you can't. It shows up in all our lives, and, since there's often not much we can do to impact the status quo that has us rushing so fast, the best possible strategy is to expect and be prepared for stress—and know how our own personal system reacts to it. This book is about maintaining an active lifestyle while you maintain your health.

Four of the five most important keys I use to maintain my health are to get plenty of sleep, get plenty of exercise, drink plenty of clean, fresh water, and fill my body with delicious, nutritious food. The fifth key is to follow a sensible program of herbs and supplements to support my body, and especially my immune system.

There are a few don'ts, too. It's best not to eat a lot of sugar or fats, not to eat just before bedtime, not to drink too much coffee or alcohol, and, of course, not to smoke or spend much time breathing polluted air. Finally, don't expect yourself to be perfect.

If a crunch time hits you, one of the worst things you can do is resort to a prescription drug.

There is plenty of well-documented research showing that popular prescribed drugs like Valium are extremely addictive and can actually increase depression. Prozac, and other antidepressant drugs in the same family (Paxil and Zoloft, for example), can cause very erratic responses in some people, including increased irritability, withdrawal from loved ones, and even violent or suicidal behavior. The side effects of these drugs are potentially so damaging that using herbal and nutritional methods to reduce anxiety and depression (which is often how we react to chronic stress) is most often the preferred method of treatment.

There are an almost infinite variety of ways that each one of us responds to stress and copes with it. Rather than using this book as a formula approach to maximizing your energy and minimizing stress, think of it as a resource with which you can discover your own personal path to an optimal high-energy lifestyle.

CHAPTER 1

Reclaiming Your Energy by Balancing Your Hormones

While your body's source of energy is food, and nutrients are transformed into energy within cells, it is certain hormones that play a vital role in regulating and synchronizing when, where and how your energy is used. When your hormones are out of balance or depleted, your energy levels can suffer. In fact, I suspect that much of what is identified as chronic fatigue syndrome is really a depletion of adrenal hormones caused by years of chronic stress.

Along with brain hormones and neurotransmitters, the steroid hormones are your most important energy regulators. They regulate and play a part in a seemingly endless list of functions in the body, including sex characteristics, sex drive, thyroid metabolism, insulin regulation, blood pressure, behavior and moods, inflammation, allergies and on and on.

The steroid hormones include those made in the adrenal glands such as cortisol and DHEA (dehydroepiandrosterone), and the sex hormones made in the ovaries and testicles such as progesterone, testosterone and estrogen. These hormones all work in synchronization with each other, and when one is depleted or excessive, it throws the rest out of balance.

All of these hormones are made in the body from cholesterol, and they all need vitamins and mineral cofactors to be produced. In other words, it takes cholesterol, plus enzymes, plus specific vitamins and minerals to produce each of the steroid hormones. Both men and women can suffer from hormone imbalance, but since women's hormones are complicated by the fact of menstrual periods, pregnancies and menopause, they tend to suffer more from imbalances.

I think that hormone replacement therapy can be very useful for many women as long as the hormones are in their natural form, and the primary hormone used is a natural progesterone cream. I've been telling you for years that synthetic hormone replacement therapy has way too many risks and side effects to be worth using, and some of the top researchers in the world continue to present evidence backing me up on this view. I'm not against hormone replacement therapy by any means. I just want you to use natural hormones, and start with the safest ones.

DON'T LET YOUR DOCTOR PUT YOU ON SYNTHETIC HORMONES

Mainstream medicine is promoting synthetic estrogens as if they will stop aging and return a woman to her youth. In fact, nothing could be further from the truth. I call estrogen the grim reaper. Estrogen in excess, or in excess relative to a shortage of progesterone, causes weight gain, bloating, headaches, irritability, depression, tender breasts, fatigue, thinning of scalp hair, foggy thinking, decreased libido, and, most life-threatening, an increased risk of strokes and cancers of the breast and reproductive organs. I believe that much fatigue in women over the age of 35 is caused by a combination of excess estrogen relative to a deficiency of progesterone, and exhausted adrenal glands.

Every risk associated with breast cancer is directly or indirectly related to estrogen, and cancers of the cervix and uterus are directly related to estrogen excess. So are fibroids, fibrocystic breasts and many of the other complaints that women have as they approach menopause.

Mainstream medicine, backed by the big drug companies, strongly pushes synthetic estrogen (Premarin, Prempro) and the synthetic progesterones called progestins (Provera, Prempro) on women of menopausal age, supposedly to reduce the risk of heart disease and osteoporosis, but the evidence for both of these claims is scanty and, as far as I'm concerned, based more on fancy juggling of statistics than reality. The fact is that estrogen will only slow bone loss for a few years around the time of menopause, and then there is no benefit. And the claims that it reduces heart disease are not only based on smoke and mirrors, the truth is that estrogen greatly raises your risk of stroke, one of the major causes of death among women.

Adding progestins to the hormone replacement mix gives some benefits, but because they are a synthetic version of progesterone, side effects include bloating, headaches, weight gain, breast tenderness and depression. Women on progestins may also suffer from migraines, asthma, breakthrough bleeding, liver damage, decreased glucose tolerance, excess hair growth, and an increased risk of stroke. Some elixir of youth!

NATURAL PROGESTERONE MAY BE YOUR ANSWER TO MENOPAUSE SYMPTOMS

Next time your doctor suggests you take Premarin or Provera for menopause, ask him or her about natural progesterone. Somehow this important hormone has been all but forgotten. And yet progesterone levels can drop to near zero at menopause, while estrogen levels only fall by 40-60 percent, just enough to stop menstrual periods and, for many women, PMS. This dramatic drop in progesterone, combined with a relatively higher level of estrogen, is responsible for most menopause symptoms.

Mainstream medicine rarely distinguishes between the synthetic progestins and natural progesterone as made by the ovaries. And yet the progestins have a long list of negative side effects, including possible miscarriage and fetal malformation, while progesterone is essential for a successful pregnancy. This alone should be a major clue to physicians and their patients that these two substances are very, very different. Sadly, very few studies have been done with progesterone, as it is a natural substance and therefore not patentable and profitable. Those that have been done show no side effects aside from some sleepiness at very high doses, and many benefits, especially for menopausal women.

Meanwhile, the latest PR/marketing salvo from the makers of Premarin, a conjugated estrogen, is that it's a "natural" hormone. Excuse me? Premarin is only natural if you're a horse. It is made from pregnant mare's urine. And those poor horses spend their lives standing in narrow stalls with catheters attached to them to collect their urine. When their foals are born they are immediately taken away (and usually killed for pet food) so the mare can be impregnated again right away. These animals suffer needlessly so the manufacturer can produce a synthetic and therefore patentable and therefore more profitable hormone, when all along the natural hormones, identical to the ones made in your body, are cheaply and easily made from plant sources.

THE HORMONE BALANCE AND ANTI-AGING SOLUTIONS FOR WOMEN

All of the maladies for which doctors are prescribing estrogen can be prevented and reversed with diet and lifestyle changes and, when necessary, with some natural progesterone cream (not the synthetic progestins), which has no side effects and all of the benefits attributed to estrogen. Some women who have persistent hot flashes and vaginal dryness may benefit from a natural estrogen cream, but most women can do just fine without it.

It is very well known now that heart disease is one of the most preventable of all chronic diseases with diet and lifestyle changes. Why should a woman increase her risk of breast cancer by 46 percent, her risk of stroke by up to 46 percent and suffer from all the estrogen and progestin side effects, when she can accomplish the same thing naturally and increase her quality of life in every way?

Women who keep their weight within reasonable limits, who keep their fat intake low and their vegetable intake high, and who get some regular exercise, rarely suffer from distressing menopause symptoms. Those who add soy products such as soy milk and tofu to their daily diet are even less likely to complain about menopause symptoms. High soy consumption and low fat consumption are almost certainly the primary reasons that hot flashes and breast cancer are virtually unknown in Japan.

Women who are at risk for osteoporosis can prevent it with a combination of diet (not too much protein, a minimum of carbonated beverages, and plenty of fresh vegetables), weight-bearing exercise and some progesterone cream, which has been convincingly shown by Dr.

John Lee to stimulate bone growth and reverse osteoporosis.

If you are a woman who is approaching menopause (i.e. over the age of 40), or menopausal, I highly recommend you read the book *What Your Doctor May Not Tell You About Menopause* by John R. Lee, M.D. (Warner Books, 1996). The book will give you an easy-to-understand yet detailed understanding of how hormone balance works, and how to balance your hormones naturally.

If your health care professional wants to test your hormone balance, I recommend the vastly less expensive and less invasive saliva hormone tests over the blood tests. They are a more accurate indicator of available hormones and are quick and easy to use. You'll find a detailed explanation of these tests and where to get them in Dr. Lee's book.

And please, do not use the "diosgenin" creams and pills touted as being a substitute for progesterone. I consider this a dangerous misconception. I know of two cases where women seeking to reverse osteoporosis with natural progesterone cream unknowingly used a diosgenin cream instead and suffered fractures because their bone density continued to decline. This is a tragic and unnecessary mistake caused by irresponsible marketing and advertising. Unfortunately, both the real progesterone creams and the diosgenin creams often identify the active ingredient as "wild yam extract," so you must know your product. The real progesterone creams generally contain about 800 milligrams of progesterone per two ounces. If you call a manufacturer to find out what's in a cream, ask directly, "Is this diosgenin or progesterone?" If the answer is that the cream does contain progesterone, ask how much. If there is under 400 mg per two ounces, find another cream.

GETTING YOUR ADRENAL GLANDS BACK IN BALANCE

As I mentioned at the beginning of this chapter, I believe that much of what is identified as chronic fatigue is really depletion and exhaustion of the adrenal glands caused by chronic stress. People who have tired adrenal glands don't have any get-up-and-go. They go to bed exhausted, wake up tired, and drag through the day trying to pump up their energy with sugar and caffeine. They gain weight because their metabolism slows down to a crawl, and they tend to complain of brain fog and muscle weakness. Their blood sugar is usually out of balance, and exercising can wipe them out for two or three days. Because the production of adrenal gland hormones is intimately tied into ovarian and testicular hormone balance, their estrogen, progesterone and testosterone levels are often way out of balance. They tend to be dizzy when they stand up suddenly, and sometimes have a rapid heartbeat when they lie down.

If this sounds like you, have your doctor check your adrenal function.

Chronic stress stimulates the release of adrenal hormones such as cortisol and adrenaline that in excess, by themselves, can throw the rest of the body's hormones out of balance. These stress hormones are designed to be released occasionally in response to extreme stress or danger, but in our fast-paced world we tend to pump them out constantly. Eventually the system breaks down, because it is not meant to be used that way.

Reducing stress, learning some type of meditation or yoga, getting plenty of sleep and rest, and eating nutritious foods will go a long way towards restoring adrenal function.

Some people with severe adrenal insufficiency may need small doses of natural hydrocortisone, which is *not* harmful, as the synthetic cortisones such as Prednisone are. For a detailed explanation of how to use hydrocortisone safely, I recommend the book *Safe Uses of Cortisone* by William McK. Jefferies, M.D. (Charles C Thomas Publisher, 1981).

SUPPLEMENTS FOR HEALTHY ADRENAL GLANDS

Many people can restore their adrenal glands and thus their energy with vitamins, minerals and herbs that nourish the adrenal glands.

Licorice root *(glycyrrhiza glabra)*, is top among herbs that support the adrenals. We think of this plant as a candy flavoring (even though most licorice candy is actually flavored with anise oil); however, the root and constituents of this herb provide a tremendous number of valuable medicinal properties.

It is a component of licorice called glycyrrhizin that stimulates the secretion of the adrenal cortex hormone aldosterone, and has a powerful cortisone-like effect. In fact, one study found that glycyrrhizin was as effective a cough suppressant as codeine, and safer. In Europe, this unique compound is used extensively for its anti-inflammatory properties, especially for Addison's disease (adrenal insufficiency) and ulcers.

Glycyrrhizin can cause high blood pressure when it is used in very high doses for many months, so some licorice preparations are de-glycyrrhizinized. This is *not* what you want if you have adrenal exhaustion. Most people with depleted adrenal glands actually have low blood pressure, so it could be just what you need! (In fact, for some, just adding more salt to the diet is enough to raise blood pressure and alleviate fatigue.)

You can take licorice root in lozenges, capsules or tincture form. Follow the directions on the container. You can increase the dose by half if it isn't having an effect. If you double the dose and it still doesn't have an effect, this may not be the herb you need.

Vitamin C is one of the most important vitamins found in the adrenal glands, and low vitamin C levels will cause lowered adrenal function. If your adrenal glands are tired, increase your vitamin C intake to bowel tolerance, which means you raise the dose until it gives you diarrhea, and then back off from that dosage level until the diarrhea goes away.

Magnesium is one of the key minerals for healthy adrenal glands because it plays an important role in regulating fluid balance in the cells, and also is an important vitamin cofactor in the manufacture of adrenal hormones. I recommend a supplement of 300-800 mg daily for supporting tired adrenals. Unbuffered magnesium can cause diarrhea, so try it in the glycinate or citrate form.

Vitamin B6 can help restore and support the adrenal glands, especially in women. Although all the B vitamins are important to healthy adrenal function, people with adrenal insufficiency are often deficient in vitamin B6. You can take 50 mg daily, in addition to your multivitamin (assuming it doesn't have more than 50 mg in it), to help replenish your adrenal glands.

Pantothenic acid (vitamin B3) directly helps strengthen the adrenal glands because it plays a role in making some of the adrenal hormones. If you're bringing your adrenal glands back up to speed, take 500-1,000 mg daily. If you're suffering from stress-induced allergies, try taking 1,000 to 2,000 mg of pantothenic acid daily.

DHEA CAN WORK WONDERS

DHEA (dehydroepiandrosterone) is an important hormone mainly made by the adrenal glands, which tends to be an androgen, or male hormone, although it is also a very important hormone for women. In both sexes DHEA is the most abundant hormone made by the adrenal glands. There is some evidence that supplementing with DHEA can reverse the drop in immune function that happens as we age.

DHEA is one of our most significant markers of aging. It begins to decline in our early twenties, and by the time we're sixty our blood levels may be almost nonexistent. In animal studies DHEA increases lifespan, lowers cholesterol, increases muscle mass and stops tumor growth. Although many claims have been made for DHEA, the single most significant factor reported in the human studies of DHEA is that even in relatively small doses people reported a greatly enhanced sense of well-being.

It is clear that some men can benefit from DHEA supplementation, as high as 100 mg a day, as they age.

There is some indication that older women may also benefit from 25 mg a day of DHEA, or 25 mg every other day, but unfortunately very little research has been done with women and DHEA. Too large a dose in women can cause male pattern baldness, insulin resistance and an increased rate of heart disease. If you are a woman, please don't take high doses of DHEA for more than a few weeks.

And please do not take diosgenin or "wild yam extract" thinking you are getting DHEA. As far as we know that doesn't happen reliably. It's best to take the real thing so you know what you're getting.

CHAPTER 2

Getting a Good Night's Sleep

Lack of sleep is one of the most common causes of fatigue, and conversely, sleep is one of the most important keys to maintaining a high-energy lifestyle. Fortunately for most people, it's relatively easy to remedy restless nights. The most obvious sleep robbers are the most common ones: stress, lack of exercise, caffeine and prescription drugs. Having to get up at night repeatedly to urinate can disturb sleeping patterns enough to cause problems. Don't drink a lot of fluids before bed, and if you're having prostate problems, use the herb saw palmetto. For details on treating prostate problems naturally, read my book *Dr. Earl Mindell's What You Should Know About Natural Health for Men* (Keats Publishing, 1996). For women, menopause may bring on hot flashes and night sweats that disturb sleep. For details on treating menopause symptoms naturally, read my book *Dr. Earl Mindell's What You Should Know About Natural Health for Women* (Keats Publishing, 1996).

DE-STRESS FOR DEEP SLEEP

Often when people are under stress and feel helpless to do anything about it, they lie awake at night tossing and turning with repetitive "tapes" going through their heads, or they wake up very early in the morning and can't get back to sleep. Big decisions, the illness or troubles of a loved one, major life changes, financial difficulties, and any number of the other lumps and bumps life hands out, can all cause sleeplessness. Depression will often cause sleeplessness, which creates a vicious circle of more depression and more sleeplessness.

There are many, many positive ways to cope with stress. One of them is to try a form of meditation that focuses on becoming aware of the mind and of your "self talk" as well as on breathing and chanting techniques which can help focus the mind. If you are unconsciously saying negative things to yourself all day long, it can be more than enough to keep you up at night! Many forms of meditation will assist you in replacing that destructive self talk with something more positive. I discuss this in more detail in the last chapter of this book.

Another way to cope with stress is to talk to a trained therapist. Just talking out loud about a problem to another human being willing to listen attentively can be enough to begin the emotional healing process. Often, when we talk about our problems out loud, resolutions begin to appear.

One technique I have found helpful when stress levels are high is to ask myself, "What is one action step I can take to reduce my stress levels?" Most often for me that step is taking a walk in a beautiful place. Sometimes it's just a matter of getting to bed earlier or spending relaxing time with my family. For some it may be a hot bath or a meal at a favorite restaurant.

More than one or two drinks of alcohol a day is not a good remedy for stress. You may escape temporarily from your problems, but excess alcohol is more likely to keep you up at night than put you to sleep, and robs your body of many nutrients.

Please don't be fooled into thinking that the new class of antidepressants such as Prozac, Paxil and Zoloft are a good solution for anything. They create a false sense of detachment and can lead to violence and suicide. Just a few of their many side effects include liver damage, depression (!) and insomnia. The companies who make these drugs are now finally being forced to admit to the FDA that they cause a withdrawal syndrome in people who stop taking them. The most common symptoms reported by people going through withdrawal are fatigue, moodiness, foggy thinking, headaches, dizziness, nausea and depression.

In ten years we will all be looking back at the "Prozac years," shaking our heads and wondering how so many people could have been so gullible to think that such drugs could be harmless. Meanwhile, countless people's lives have already been destroyed by them. Even though they are being handed out like candy by many doctors, I urge you to resist the urge to change your personality with a pill. First try a balanced, moderate lifestyle, cutting down on stress, getting some exercise, plenty of sleep and some nutritional supplements, which I'll cover later in the book.

EXERCISE CAN BE A SIMPLE, EFFECTIVE CURE FOR INSOMNIA

Exercise is by far my favorite sleeping pill and cure for the blues. I have seen many people suffering from mild depression or insomnia cure it simply by getting some exercise. Somehow we resist the simple cures to our problems, but exercise is one of your best bets for a good night's sleep. A brisk 20- to 30-minute walk daily can be just the sleeping potion you need.

As for maintaining peak energy, anyone who exercises regularly knows that you use energy or lose it. Working the body keeps its fuel systems active, bringing in oxygen used to burn the calories taken in from food, which produces energy. Energy is needed for every activity, even sleeping. When you have optimum fitness you'll have optimum energy. The greater the energy, the more active you can be in every area of your life and the better you'll function on every level, including physical, mental and emotional.

IS CAFFEINE YOUR SLEEP ROBBER?

Too much caffeine, or caffeine too late in the day can keep your eyes wide open for hours into the night. While this might be nice if you're working a night shift, for most of us it only leads to bleary eyes and fatigue the next day. Some people are so sensitive to caffeine that a cup of coffee any time after noon will keep them awake at night. And let's not forget that green tea and black tea contain caffeine, and even decaf still contains some caffeine. If you're suffering from insomnia, your best bet is to drink non-stimulating herbal teas such as chamomile or mint in the evening. If you need a boost in the afternoon, try a cup of ginseng tea.

ARE YOUR MEDICATIONS KEEPING YOU UP?

Many over-the-counter pain killers, cold and allergy remedies and appetite suppressants contain caffeine and other substances that can cause insomnia. Some examples are Anacin, Extra Strength Excedrin, Bayer Select Maximum, Midol and Vanquish.

Allergy and cold medicines may contain synthetic variations of ephedrine, such as pseudoephedrine (Sudafed), which can keep you awake. The asthma drug theophylline (Bronkaid and Primatene tablets, Tedral and others) are stimulants that can make sleeping difficult.

The cortisones, such as Prednisone, can also cause sleeplessness. The heart drugs such as propranolol, furosemide and lovastatin may cause insomnia, as can too high a dose of thyroid medication such as Synthroid. Ironically, many of the antidepressants cause insomnia, which can cause depression due to lack of sleep!

Unfortunately, if one of these medications is keeping you awake at night, your doctor is most likely to write you out a prescription for a sleeping pill. In nearly all cases, that is the worst possible thing you can do for insomnia. Sleeping pills cause either dependence or outright addiction very quickly, they tend to lose their effectiveness over time, and have a rebound effect if you stop, causing worse insomnia than ever. They also tend to suppress your dream or REM sleep, sometimes resulting in severe mental disturbances and psychoses if used over a long period of time. If someone hands you a prescription for a sleeping pill, my advice is to run the other way.

If you're having trouble sleeping and taking any type of medication, including over-the-counter drugs, read the label or package insert to find out if it can cause insomnia, restlessness or irritability.

SUPPLEMENTS FOR SLEEP

A variety of supplements can help you sleep at night. A deficiency of B vitamins, calcium or magnesium can keep you awake. As we age, our production of melatonin, a hormone that regulates sleep-wake cycles, declines. A simple melatonin supplement may be your ticket to a good night's sleep if you're a senior citizen.

The B Vitamins

The B vitamins together and separately play important roles in nerve and brain function and in relaxing muscles. If you are older and not absorbing nutrients as well as you might be, your body may not be able to utilize the B vitamins in your food. It's important to include the B vitamins in a multivitamin. If you're having trouble with leg cramps at night, an extra 50 mg of vitamin B6 an hour before bed may help. I have heard many anecdotal stories of people curing restless leg syndrome by taking an extra 400 mcg of folic acid before bed.

Calcium and Magnesium

Both of these important minerals play a role in muscle relaxation, the prevention of muscle spasms, and the balance of fluid in the cells. If you tend to tense up physically when you're under stress, or if you suffer from leg cramps at night, calcium and magnesium might be the supplements for you. These two supplements should be taken together, since calcium can't do many of its jobs in the body without magnesium. You can take 600-800 mg of calcium and 300-600 mg of magnesium about an hour before bedtime. There are many formulas that combine these two minerals in a ratio of 2:1 calcium to magnesium, and these are fine.

Using Melatonin to Improve Sleep

Melatonin is a safe, effective, natural sleep remedy that is free of side effects when used as directed. It is normally secreted by the brain in response to darkness.

Since it regulates sleep-wake cycles, melatonin

can also be very useful for banishing jet lag by adjusting circadian rhythms to match your geographic location. You do this simply by taking melatonin about an hour before you want to sleep in your new location. It will give your brain the message that it's time to sleep, regardless of what time zone you're in. One or two nights of melatonin should put you back on the right track.

As for the claims that melatonin is an anti-aging drug, we need to be cautious in making the leap from extending lifespan in a particular strain of mice to extending lifespan in humans. In some studies mice that were given melatonin lived 20 percent longer, but other strains of mice in other studies died sooner. Younger mice given melatonin developed cancer, and melatonin in high doses suppresses sex hormones.

While I use melatonin regularly when I travel, to erase jet lag, and recommend it for older people who are having trouble sleeping, I want to caution you that we simply don't know the long-term effects of using melatonin every night. Any time we take a hormone in higher doses than the body would naturally produce, we're asking for an imbalance.

If you are over the age of 65 and your melatonin levels have dropped so far that you can't sleep at night, *and* you have eliminated other possible causes of your insomnia, then by all means, take 0.5 to 3 mg at night to help you sleep. In that case, you are correcting a deficiency. It is also perfectly safe to take melatonin for an occasional bout of insomnia. Melatonin is a natural hormone, so when it is used occasionally your body should have no trouble excreting any excess.

If you need melatonin, it only takes a very small dose to help you sleep better. If low melatonin levels aren't your problem, even a big dose won't make any difference.

The melatonin sold in health food stores is manufactured, but is the exact molecular structure as the melatonin made by the body. Sublingual forms of melatonin are more expensive but act more quickly. Look for a reputable brand at your health food store. Take melatonin tablets about one hour before you want to go to sleep, and the sublingual tablets half an hour before you want to go to sleep.

Some drugs, including NSAIDs (nonsteroidal anti-inflammatory drugs such as aspirin, ibuprofen and acetaminophen), interfere with the brain's production of melatonin. In fact, just one dose of normal aspirin can cut your melatonin production as much as 75 percent. If you're taking these drugs, take the last dose after dinner. Other drugs that can interfere with melatonin production in the brain include the benzodiazepines such as Valium and Xanax, caffeine, alcohol, cold medicines, diuretics, beta blockers, calcium-channel blockers, stimulants such as diet pills, and corticosteroids such as Prednisone.

TRYPTOPHAN MAY HELP YOU SLEEP

The amino acid tryptophan, a precursor to melatonin, is a very safe and effective sleep remedy, and can also be a wonderful remedy for anxiety and depression. Unfortunately it was pulled off the market in the U.S. by the FDA when a contaminated batch from Japan made some people ill. This type of contamination could have happened in thousands of drugs, and the illness it caused had nothing to do with the effects of uncontaminated tryptophan. In truth, tryptophan is very safe—in my opinion it is far safer than sleeping pills and antidepressants, which it was competing with in a big way when it was pulled off the market. My guess is that tryptophan was removed from the market to protect the profits of the big drug companies, not to protect your health.

Tryptophan's effect on the brain is similar to that of drugs such as Prozac, except that it doesn't have the side effects and dangers and withdrawal problems those drugs have, it's much less expensive, and it's probably more effective. Tryptophan is trickling back onto the market in the U.S., and it can be purchased almost anywhere outside the United States.

One of tryptophan's primary effects on the brain is to reduce anxiety, which is often the culprit in insomnia. However, even if tryptophan is unavailable where you live, there are some herbs that can work wonders to alleviate feelings of anxiety.

GETTING A GOOD NIGHT'S SLEEP

CALMING HERBS

The herbs I recommend most often for treating depression and anxiety are St. John's wort and kava.

St. John's wort, which has been used successfully for many centuries by the Chinese, the Greeks, the Europeans and the American Indians, is well known for its positive effect on anxiety, insomnia, depression, and a physical illness which has long been associated with stress: heart disease.

St. John's wort, which you can get easily both as a tincture and in capsule form at your health food store, has no known side effects in humans. (If grazing cattle eat huge amounts of fresh St. John's wort, they have been found to develop photosensitivity, but so far I've heard no reports of humans having this problem—and humans would be highly unlikely to eat a proportionate amount of St. John's wort or to eat it fresh.) These positive effects are even more positive when weighed against even the less dramatic side effects of pharmaceutical drugs like drowsiness, constipation and dry mouth.

Take it in the dose recommended on the container.

Kava is one of our most useful antianxiety herbs. Anyone who's been to the South Pacific, where it grows like a bush, has probably tried it. Its Latin name is *Piper methysticum,* and it's a member of the pepper family. Kava is described medically as a sedative and muscle relaxant. It's also a pain reliever, often working just as well as NSAIDs (drugs in the aspirin, ibuprofen and acetaminophen family).

As a folk medicine, kava is attributed with the power to bring on well-being and to encourage socializing. Many studies, mostly done in Europe, have demonstrated how effective kava is in the treatment of anxiety and depression. It has worked as effectively as benzodiazepines, of which Valium, Librium and Serax are examples. In many ways, kava's effects are preferable. Rather than causing lethargy, drowsiness and mental impairment (which are common responses to benzodiazepines) kava improves concentration, memory and reaction time for people with anxiety symptoms. And the best part is, no side effects have been noted, except with very large amounts taken over a number of years. However, kava is not recommended for people with Parkinson's or Alzheimer's disease.

Kava is best taken powdered in a capsule or as a liquid extract. Follow the directions on the container.

CHAPTER 3

Supplements for a Strong Immune System

The immune system, which protects us from harmful bacteria, viruses, fungi and other so-called "foreign invaders," makes its presence known in every system of the body.

Unlike the circulatory system, or the reproductive system, you can't see the immune system on an anatomy chart or remove it in surgery, and yet it is equivalent in its size and daily activity to a large organ that produces billions of new cells each day. It rallies its defenses from the cellular level, everywhere in the body, from deep within the brain and bone marrow, to the adrenal glands, the thymus gland and the skin. It courses through the blood and the intestines; its wastes are dumped into the lymphatic system, the kidneys and the liver for detoxifying, and it relies on an intricate identification system to discriminate between the good guys and the bad guys. When this identification system goes awry we get autoimmune diseases and allergies. We fall prey to infections, viral diseases and cancers when we are unable to rally the vast armies of specialized cells designed to protect us from deadly threats we can't see. These immune cells go by such names as white blood cells, T cells, helper cells, lymphocytes and macrophages.

Without a healthy immune system it is impossible to lead a fully active, healthy life. Keeping the immune system on full alert and in balance is achieved by keeping all levels in balance—physical, emotional, mental and spiritual. Our immune system balance is intricately tied into our thoughts and emotions, as well as nutrition, exercise and environmental toxins.

All nutrients are important to the immune system, and have a direct effect on it. A study in Newfoundland found that senior citizens who consumed a multivitamin supplement for one year had many increased immune responses and fewer days of illness due to infectious diseases. Let's zero in on those vitamins that affect your immune system the most.

Vitamin A is important in maintaining the integrity of the skin and mucous membranes, your front-line defenses against airborne and intestinal invaders. Your largest mucous membrane is in the intestines, which contain a wide variety of immune cells. Vitamin A has been shown to stimulate many immune processes. It helps fight infection, is antiviral, and anticarcinogenic. A large supplemental dose of vitamin A can reverse the suppression of the immune system that occurs after surgery, and improves wound healing. On a day-to-day basis you can get most of your vitamin A from carotenoids such as beta-carotene, from which the body will make vitamin A as needed.

In a study with AIDS patients, beta-carotene in doses of 180 International Units created an increase in helper cells. If you are fighting an infection or a virus, you can take up to 50,000 IU of vitamin A daily for 3-5 days, then 25,000 IU daily for a week or two. Since vitamin A accumulates in the body and can be toxic in high doses, it's best not to take it in high doses for more than a few weeks. Pregnant women shouldn't take more than 10,000 IU of vitamin A in supplement form daily.

The B vitamins are essential immune system boosters. Both vitamin B12 and folic acid play a particularly important role in the production of white blood cells and lymphocyte response. Population studies show an association between low levels of folic acid (folate) and cancer of the cervix, colon, lung, esophagus and brain. According to Dr. John Lee in his new book, *What Your Doctor May Not Tell You About Menopause* (Warner Books, 1996), folic acid supplementation can reverse precancerous growth of the cervix called cervical dysplasia.

You should be getting 200 mcg of folic acid daily in supplement form, up to 600 mcg daily if you are battling illness and at least 400 mcg daily if there is any possibility you could become pregnant. (Folic acid deficiencies can cause birth defects.)

Since vitamin B12 is not well absorbed when it is taken orally, you can take it in the form of a nasal gel or sublingually (under the tongue), 1,000 mcg one to three times daily when you need a boost.

Pantothenic acid (vitamin B5) supports adrenal and pituitary hormones and reduces the body's histamine response. Take at least 25 mg daily, and up to 100 mg if your immune system needs to shift into high gear. Low vitamin B6 levels have been found to correlate with a low T cell counts. In one eight-week study, 50 mg of vitamin B6 per day stimulated lymphocytes. Take 50 mg daily, and up to 100 mg when stress levels are high. This vitamin is particularly important for maintaining hormone balance in women who are under stress.

Vitamin C is a primary weapon in the immune system's arsenal against bacteria and viruses. When you need an extra boost to your immune system from vitamin C, try taking 1,500 to 4,000 mg in a buffered powder form that includes calcium, magnesium and potassium. At the same time you take the vitamin C, take a bioflavonoid supplement, which will maximize your body's use of the vitamin C.

Vitamin E is one of the superstars of the vitamin world when it comes to boosting the immune system. Studies show that it increases helper T cells and antibody response, both potent weapons of the immune system. A study of vitamin E with healthy people taking 800 IU per day, showed that it enhanced immune responses. When you're looking for an immune system boost, take 800 IU daily of d-alpha tocopherol. For maximum absorption, take it in the dry or "succinate" form.

Probiotics, particularly *Lactobacillus acidophilus*, are "good" intestinal bacteria that support the immune system by bringing the intestinal flora into balance. *Prebiotics* are nondigestible "food" for probiotics, but not for harmful bacteria. Fructooligosaccharides

(FOS) are prebiotics that are now included in many probiotic products. I recommend you choose a probiotic-prebiotic combination that is dated and refrigerated. Follow the directions on the container.

Dehydroepiandrosterone (DHEA), which we looked at in relationship to hormonal balance in Chapter 1, is an adrenal hormone that declines with age, and any type of illness involving adrenal insufficiency. Studies have found low DHEA levels in people who have AIDS and leukemia, and some researchers theorize that the hormone plays an important role in regulating T cells. This can be a very useful supplement for those suffering from chronic illness who have low levels of DHEA, or for people over the age of 50. Women should keep their dosage low, up to 20-25 mg daily or every other day, as DHEA is an androgen, or masculinizing hormone. Men can take up to 100 mg daily, but 50 mg is the usual maintenance dose.

Minerals are essential components of a healthy immune system, and you should be getting them every day in a multivitamin. A deficiency of minerals such as zinc and selenium can lead to reduced cellular immunity and an increased susceptibility to infection. Selenium deficiency is common in AIDS and colon cancer patients, people with chronic diarrhea, and those with poor absorption of nutrients. Deficiencies of selenium and zinc can indicate a depressed immune system. One way selenium supports the immune system is by acting as an antioxidant, mopping up free radicals that damage cells. Zinc deficiency causes the thymus, one of our primary immune system organs, to shrink.

Low zinc levels also cause poor wound healing, decreased numbers of T cells, lymphocytes and natural killer cells. Zinc works with Vitamin A to maintain mucous membranes, and is especially important in fighting off viruses. Iron deficiency can result in a decrease in T cell-mediated immunity.

Manganese increases natural killer cell activity. It is depleted from most soils, so this is an important trace mineral to include in a daily multivitamin.

Essential fatty acids (EFAs), oils found primarily in vegetables, nuts, seeds, fish, flax seed oil, evening primrose oil and borage oil, affect the balance of prostaglandins, hormone-like substances that play an important role in regulating the immune system. Supplementing AIDS and cancer patients with omega-3 fatty acids (fish oils, flax seed oil, evening primrose oil) has been shown to improve a depressed immune system. Other studies have shown that fish oil supplementation has an anti-inflammatory effect, inhibits tumor growth and speeds healing after surgery.

Linoleic acid, an omega-6 fatty acid found in many vegetable oils, is necessary for T cells to work properly. On the other hand, too high an intake of linoleic acid, especially relative to not enough omega-3 fatty acids, will suppress immune function. This may be useful in treating autoimmune diseases, but some researchers believe that the increase in consumption of polyunsaturated oils such as vegetable oils and margarines has contributed to the increase in asthma and other lung-related problems over the past three decades, by blocking "good" prostaglandin pathways.

Glutamine is the most abundant free amino acid in the human body. While glutamine is not considered an essential amino acid because your body can make plenty of it under normal circumstances, it becomes essential when you're under physical stress. It plays a powerful and essential role in maintaining a healthy digestive system, a strong immune system, in muscle strength and in the chemical balance of the brain. Some researchers believe glutamine is *the* most essential nutrient in the digestive tract. When you're under stress, particularly stress caused by surgery, illness or injury, the levels of glutamine in your body can drop up to 90 percent.

Studies have shown that surgery patients who are given supplemental glutamine after surgery recover faster and have a shorter hospital stay. Glutamine has also been shown in animal studies to enhance the tumor-killing effects of chemotherapy and radiation, and to reduce their side effects.

Glutamine is not recommended if you have severe liver disease or other illnesses that could involve an accumulation of ammonia in the blood. I recommend you take this supplement in the L-glutamine form, as a powder, capsule or tablets.

Glutathione is an antioxidant made in the body by three amino acids, cysteine, glycine and glutamic acid. Its primary job is neutralizing and disposing of free radicals, in coordination with vitamin E and vitamin C. It's also crucial in protecting the lymphatic system, one of the body's primary weapons in fighting infection. Glutathione directly improves immune function and protects the body against free radicals and external toxins. If glutathione levels drop anywhere in the body, the burden of toxic stress goes up. T cells cannot function when glutathione levels are low.

Glutathione concentrations are high in healthy people. People with chronic conditions such as heart disease, arthritis and diabetes have low glutathione levels. The best way to raise glutathione levels is by taking a cysteine supplement, 500 to 1,000 mg daily (the body uses cysteine to make glutathione). You can take it in the form of cysteine or N-acetyl cysteine.

Echinacea is an herb that acts as a powerful immune system booster. It can be very useful in preventing colds and flus or in shortening their duration. Don't take echinacea for more than two weeks at a time, or it will start to lose its effectiveness.

10 MORE NATURAL WAYS TO CHARGE UP YOUR IMMUNE SYSTEM

1. Stretching helps your lymphatic system do its job of removing toxins from your body. Chi gong is an especially effective form of exercise for boosting the immune system.

2. Take a good multivitamin. (Read my book in this series, *Earl Mindell's What You Should Know About Creating Your Personal Vitamin Plan,* Keats Publishing 1996.)

3. Exercise keeps everything in the body shipshape, but if you feel weak or tired, don't push it too hard, it will only make things worse. If you have a cold or flu you need rest.

4. Drink plenty of clean water which will help your body keep itself detoxified.

5. Eat plenty of fiber to keep things moving through the digestive system.

6. Eat yogurt once a day for the calcium and beneficial intestinal flora. The friendly bacteria in your intestines are your best weapon against unfriendly bacteria.

7. Eat your vegetables—fresh and preferably organic. And I'm not talking iceberg lettuce here, I'm talking the real stuff like carrots, broccoli, spinach and beets.

8. Eat more complex carbohydrates and less refined white flour which causes blood sugar jumps and constipation.

9. Try shiitake or reishi mushrooms with your veggies—the Chinese use them to bolster the immune system.

10. If you have a late night or stressful day, balance things out by getting extra rest.

CHAPTER 4

Are Allergies Bringing You Down?

Spring is a fresh, exuberant time of year, with balmy breezes, green grass sprouting, and flowers blooming everywhere. But if you have allergies to pollens and grasses, as one in ten Americans does, spring may only mean fatigue, mental fogginess, sniffling, snuffling and sneezing to you. The normal response to allergy symptoms is to take drugs such as antihistamines, but as most of us have discovered, they all have undesirable side effects.

Allergies in general can also be caused by food, food additives and dyes, chemical sprays and fumes, dust, pet hair and fleas, molds, medication, perfumes, cosmetics, feathers and dozens of other environmental offenders. While avoiding the offender works in part, it is also important to support your immune system.

WHY DO WE SNEEZE AND SNIFFLE?

We get allergies to pollen when our immune system is reacting, or sensitive, to something in the environment that is actually harmless. It's helpful (if not pleasant!) when our bodies fight off a real invader such as a virus or bacteria with an immune reaction, which we call a cold or flu. But when we react to pollens, it's annoying and can interfere with our enjoyment of life.

Once our immune system decides that a particular type of pollen is a hostile invader, it becomes "sensitized" to it, and can react with allergy symptoms for years, and perhaps a lifetime. When spring arrives and the pollen begins to fly, our sensitized bodies release histamines, designed to fight the enemy pollen. In the process of attacking the invaders, the histamines cause inflammation and even damage tissues, causing sinus irritation, itchy eyes and often lung irritation as well. Some people may even develop rashes, eczema or hives.

The frequent accompanying headaches and mental fogginess are caused by sinus congestion. Sneezing is caused by irritated sinuses. Sore throats are caused by the mucus that runs down the back of the throat. Asthma can be triggered by an overload of irritants and mucus. If the body tries to rid itself of the invaders via the skin, rashes, eczema and hives may result.

Allergy drugs work to suppress symptoms rather than treat the cause of the allergy. The consequences of this type of treatment are generally unpleasant side effects and often a rebound effect where the symptom is worse if the medication starts to wear off or treatment is stopped.

NATURAL REMEDIES FOR ALLERGIES

The simplest way to avoid allergy symptoms is to avoid the offending allergens, but if you're allergic to pollens and grasses, yet love the outdoors and fresh air, this isn't a practical solution. The next simplest way to deal with allergies is to drink plenty of clean water. I recommend at least 8-10 glasses a day during allergy season. Water not only helps flush toxins out of the body and supports proper cell function, but as our water levels go down, our histamine levels go up. Drinking a couple of glasses of clean water can quickly reduce allergy symptoms.

The reason some people suffer from allergies and others don't certainly has to do with genetic predispositions, but also seems to have to do with how well your immune system is working. If you already have a weakened immune system from chronic nutritional deficiencies, disease, lack of exercise or other factors, you're much more susceptible to allergies.

Echinacea is a powerful immune system booster. Take two droppersful of the tincture (preferably the fresh extract) in water, or two capsules, three times daily. Don't take echinacea for more than two weeks at a time, or it will start to lose its effectiveness. Through allergy season, take it two weeks on and two weeks off.

Astragalus: This Chinese plant has been used by healers in that country for centuries to restore normal function to the immune system. Follow the directions on the container.

Shiitake and reishi mushrooms are another Oriental remedy for the immune system. I like them best in a vegetable stir-fry or in an omelet! They're expensive, but you don't need to use much—one or two small mushrooms per serving should do the trick. During allergy season add these to your diet at least once a week, or take them in capsule form.

Garlic: The more we study and research garlic, the better it looks. If you like the taste, make it a part of your daily diet; and if you don't, you can take it in capsule form. In addition to lowering cholesterol levels and blood pressure, killing intestinal parasites, reducing the risk of blood clots, inhibiting some cancer tumors and aiding digestion, garlic is a potent antioxidant, helping the body keep our cells healthy, intact and functioning smoothly.

Yogurt: If you eat yogurt with live cultures daily as I recommend, you may greatly reduce the severity of your seasonal allergy symptoms. A one-year study at the University of California at Davis showed that those who ate just under a cup of yogurt daily had significantly reduced hay fever symptoms as well as fewer colds. Dr. Halpern, who did the study, found that two cups of yogurt a day worked even better than one.

Ephedra (also called Mormon Tea and ma huang): This plant contains ephedrine. Pseudoephedrine is the synthetic version of ephedrine, and is commonly found in over-the-counter allergy drugs. It is widely used in diet pills because it's an "upper." However, the downside, as I mentioned above, is that it can also make you "hyper" or restless, irritable, nervous, and can cause insomnia. While it is effective in reducing the symptoms of congestion, I urge you not to use it over a long period of time. Please work on the underlying causes of your allergies first, and take the steps I recommend, reserving these types of drugs for occasional symptomatic use. Please don't use ephedra at all if you have high blood pressure or heart disease.

Milk thistle *(Silybum marianum)*: This is one of the hot "new" herbs that's been used in folk medicine for centuries and is now gaining respectability thanks to scientific studies. It has been clearly shown in studies to greatly support the liver, even to the extent of regenerating liver cells. Since your liver is one of the main places your immune system dumps toxins, it pays to support it during allergy season. Take one capsule three times daily. Make sure your milk thistle product is taken from the seeds, which contain the most of the active ingredient, silymarin. These seeds are also rich in linoleic acid, which supports the production of prostaglandins, another important hormone-like substance. Linoleic acid also appears to help regulate the female hormones.

VITAMINS AND MINERALS THAT HELP WITH ALLERGIES

Vitamin C: If I could only recommend one vitamin to help with allergy symptoms it would be vitamin C. This essential vitamin, which many Americans are deficient in, works directly to lower histamine levels in the body and supports the immune system in many ways. During allergy season I recommend you take at least 1,000 mg three times daily; and if your symptoms continue or get worse, increase that to 1,000 mg every two or three hours.

Quercetin: This is a powerful antioxidant flavonoid that has been shown to fight cancer tumors and seems to be very effective in helping fight allergy symptoms. I like it combined with bromelain for better absorption.

Grapeseed Extract: The star of the antioxidant world is a complex of substances called proanthocyanidins, known for short as PCOs. I like the PCOs extracted from grapeseeds. They rank among our most powerful flavonoids, being 50 times more powerful at scavenging free radicals than vitamin E, and 20 times more powerful than vitamin C. Furthermore, they enhance the potency of both these vitamins.

You can take 150-300 mg of PCOs daily to combat allergies. I recommend the grapeseed PCO extract that comes in a "phytosome" package, meaning the molecules are combined with phosphatidylcholine, a natural component of lecithin. This new process allows the body to absorb and utilize much more of the PCO than it would otherwise.

OTHER ALLERGY REMEDIES

Homeopathic remedies: There are dozens of homeopathic remedies for allergies, with very specific applications. If you want to try that route, I recommend you read the books *Everybody's Guide to Homeopathic Medicine*, by Stephen Cummings and Dana Ullman, (Jeremy Tarcher), *Homeopathic Medicine at Home* by Panos and Heimlich (Jeremy Tarcher) or *The Family Guide to Homeopathy* by Dr. Andrew Locke (Simon & Schuster Fireside). For more in-depth treatment, find an experienced homeopathic physician.

Ping Chuan Pill: This is a Chinese patent medicine that can be very helpful in supporting the immune system and reducing symptoms. However, since it does treat symptoms, I don't recommend using it on a long-term basis.

CHAPTER 5

Boosting Energy and Brain Power Naturally

The most important thing you can do for your brain is to feed it well, which is the same as feeding the rest of your body. Everything you eat affects your brain to some extent. I can't emphasize enough how important a healthy lifestyle is to a healthy brain. Brain function is dependent on balanced nutrition, and particularly on keeping your body's detoxification systems working effectively. The additives, preservatives and dyes found in processed food only add to your body's detoxification load. Your body will have less to detoxify if you're careful about what you put in it.

Clean water is your most important detoxifier, and exercise is your second most important detoxifier.

Your brain needs plenty of B vitamins to function properly, it needs amino acids, stable blood sugar, and it needs plenty of oxygen. The brain also needs glucose in abundance. Glucose is a sugar the body makes from the foods we eat. It is the primary source of energy for the brain. Your brain literally cannot function without it. If your glucose or blood sugar levels remain relatively stable, your brain will work better. That means keeping your weight down, avoiding sweets and other refined foods, and getting some exercise.

Exercise improves circulation, increasing your oxygen supply to the brain via better blood flow. Glucose and oxygen work together in the brain. If your blood isn't getting enough oxygen, your brain won't work as well. Exercise is one of the best ways to increase blood flow to the brain.

PREVENTING MEMORY LOSS AND BRAIN FOG

If glucose is the energy source for the brain, a substance called glutamate is the mainstay of the communications systems of the brain. Glutamate is a brain "excitor," meaning it excites brain cells into action. With the proper balance of glutamate, your brain functions well. Too little glutamate is rarely a problem. However, if the brain gets too much glutamate, the brain cells excite themselves to death and if it continues, you lose brain function, starting with memory.

Glutamate is probably a familiar word to you because you've heard of monosodium glutamate, or MSG. Millions of pounds of MSG are dumped in our food every year, much to the detriment of our brain health. Since MSG has gotten a bad reputation, food manufacturers, ever alert to increasing profits at the expense of your health, have learned to disguise MSG on labels by calling it natural flavoring, hydrolyzed vegetable protein, vegetable protein, and spices (while the FDA looks the other way). New labeling laws were supposed to mandate that all MSG-type products be labeled as glutamate, but somehow they got lost in the political maze of the FDA. The best way to avoid glutamate is to avoid processed foods and be discriminating about eating in restaurants.

Glutamate has a close cousin called aspartate, another brain excitor which also has important functions in brain communications. Aspartate should be familiar to you as a part of the artificial sweetener aspartame, otherwise known as NutraSweet. Test animals fed MSG and aspartate, even in low doses over a long period of time, end up with symptoms identical to Alzheimer's. If you want to keep your memory powered up for life, I urge you to avoid these substances. This means avoiding refined foods, diet sodas, and other artificially sweetened foods and drinks. There's no doubt that MSG and all its relatives make food tastier, but who wants to sacrifice brain cells and memory!

The amino acid glutamine is closely related to glutamate, but when you take it as a supplement your body can either turn it into glutamine as needed, or into other related amino acids.

Brain fog can have many causes, or a combination of causes. Some of the most common are unstable blood sugar, excess estrogen, low thyroid, exhausted adrenal glands, and lack of sleep. Another very common cause of brain fog is pollen allergies, which are covered in this book, and food allergies and sensitivities, which are covered in my book *Dr. Earl Mindell's What You Should Know About Fiber and Digestion* (Keats, 1996).

If you are sensitive to environmental toxins and irritants such as car exhaust, pesticides, fumes from newly painted rooms or new carpets, solvents, scented laundry soaps, fabric softeners and perfumes, your brain can "crash" just from exposure to these substances. If this describes you, your best approach is to make every effort to avoid exposure to such substances while building up your immune system as much as possible. I recommend working with a health-care professional knowledgeable in alternative medicine if you have environmental sensitivities.

IS YOUR PRESCRIPTION FOGGING YOUR BRAIN?

If you're taking prescription drugs, please keep in mind that many of them can cause memory loss and brain fog. The most common types of drugs that can cause memory loss are the ulcer drugs such as Tagamet and Zantac; the high blood pressure drugs such as beta blockers and diuretics; and the antidepressants, antipsychotics, barbiturates, sleeping pills and tranquilizers such as Prozac, Nembutal, Atarax, Dalmane and Valium.

Remember, keeping your memory powered up for life is mainly a matter of a healthy lifestyle. If you supply your brain with a good environment, it will supply you with a good memory.

Sometimes during times of stress or illness, or as we age, we need some help powering up the brain. Here are some natural ways to boost your brain power and at the same time, your energy.

MEMORY BOOSTERS

Ginkgo biloba: This is one of my favorite memory boosters because it's very effective, very safe, and not expensive. It's been extensively researched, and is sold in standardized amounts, so you know what you're getting.

The ginkgo biloba tree has been on this planet longer than any other species of tree. It has been around for at least 300 million years! The Chinese have been using ginkgo medicinally for at least 5,000 years.

Ginkgo has been shown over and over again in top-notch research studies done in Europe to be very effective in treating what is called in medical circles "cerebral insufficiency," or impaired blood flow to the brain. It can improve the ability to remember, the speed of memory and mental performance, as well as relieving symptoms of cerebral insufficiency such as headaches, dizziness, ringing in the ears, clumsiness and hearing impairment.

Ginkgo may be one of our most important anti-aging medicines. If you're over the age of 60 I recommend you take it daily as health insurance. It may be a few weeks before you notice results.

The best way to take ginkgo is in a liquid extract, capsules or tablets that are at least 24 percent ginkgo flavoglycosides.

Acetylcholine is a neurotransmitter, meaning it is a chemical that transfers messages from one brain cell to another. When those messages are disrupted by a lack of acetylcholine, or less effective acetylcholine receptors in the brain cells, symptoms such as memory loss and confused thinking can result. Researchers at the University of California have theorized that one of the causes of Alzheimer's disease is a destruction of the cells that supply acetylcholine to the parts of the brain involved in memory and cognitive thinking. When they increased acetylcholine levels in the brains of rats with brain damage equivalent to Alzheimer's, they found they could restore their memory.

In another study done at Hebrew University, a research team discovered that memory loss could be caused simply by an excess of a brain enzyme called acetylcholinesterase, which breaks down acetylcholine.

Increasing your brain's supply of acetylcholine is a safe, natural way to give your brain what it needs to do the job. If you are taking anticholinergic drugs to treat Parkinson's disease, you won't want to use supplements that boost acetylcholine. One of the other jobs acetylcholine has in the body is to make your muscles contract. Anticholinergic drugs are used in Parkinson's and in some digestive tract diseases to reduce muscle contraction. The next four supplements listed will help you build your acetylcholine levels.

Pantothenic acid (vitamin B5 or pantothenate) acts as an enzyme that builds the acetylcholine molecule. Take 200—500 mg daily.

Phosphatidylcholine (the active ingredient in lecithin) is a building block for acetylcholine. You can take it as a liquid, as a capsule, or as 1 tablespoon daily of lecithin granules that can sprinkled on cereal or other foods or just eaten plain. Be sure the lecithin is at least 55 percent phosphatidylcholine, and be sure that it is fresh, not rancid. It should have a pleasant, nutty smell and taste. Since choline increases the secretion of stomach acid, this may be helpful if your digestion is poor; but if you have ulcers, please wait until they're healed before using choline. Take 1,500—2,500 mg daily.

Niacin (niacinamide, vitamin B3) is a cofactor in building acetylcholine. Take 50-100 mg of niacin in the form of niacinamide, daily. If you are experiencing flushing, take it with a meal. With this small a dose, flushing usually goes away after a week or two.

Glutamic acid is a brain-stimulating amino acid that may increase the number of acetylcholine receptor sites in your brain cells. It is the amino acid found in the highest concentration in the brain after aspartate, and the brain spends a great deal of energy keeping it balanced with its close relatives glutamine and gamma-aminobutyric acid (GABA). It can also be made into glutamate, which may sound familiar from the flavor-enhancer monosodium glutamate (MSG), a highly absorbable and easily toxic form of glutamic acid. Because glutamate in excess can become a brain toxin, I want you to take this amino acid in the form of glutamine, which the body will easily convert to whichever form it needs in the brain without toxicity. If you have cancer, do not take glutamine, as it can act as a food for cancerous tumors. Take 500-1,000 mg daily.

Carnitine is a nonessential amino acid that can become essential if your brain isn't functioning as well as it could. Although carnitine is not an essential amino acid, meaning that our bodies can synthesize it, a deficiency can cause fatigue, muscle weakness, heart disease, acidic blood, high triglyceride levels and brain degeneration. Taking carnitine as a supplement can enhance the body's ability to burn fat, prevent heart disease and improve brain deterioration as we age.

We get carnitine in meat and we make it from lysine, which is found in whole grains, legumes such as soy, and meats. To manufacture carnitine, the body also needs vitamin B6, niacin, iron, and vitamin C.

It's only been recently that researchers have made advances in understanding how carnitine affects the brain. Current theory is that carnitine enhances brain function by improving the energy levels of brain cells by transporting fats across cell membranes into the mitochondria. In one double-blind, placebo-controlled study of carnitine, 30 mildly to moderately demented patients with probable Alzheimer's disease were randomly assigned to receive either carnitine or a placebo. After 6 months, the treated group showed significantly less brain deterioration. This is just one of several recently published studies showing similar results. No pharmaceutical drug has shown these kinds of results! Carnitine is already being used extensively in Italy to treat brain deterioration.

And you don't need to have a failing memory to benefit from carnitine. A study done in Italy of healthy people showed that after 30 days of carnitine supplementation they were better able to pay attention, had faster reflexes, and better eye-hand coordination. Other studies have shown that carnitine supplementation improves long-term memory, increases alertness and improves learning ability. In every study, a certain percentage of people also report improved mood. Carnitine's ability to protect brain neurons and enhance their responsiveness also makes it one of our most important anti-aging supplements.

Carnitine comes in several forms at your health food store. The forms I recommend are either L-carnitine, acetyl L-carnitine, or L-acetylcarnitine. The acetylated forms may help absorption, but they also tend to be more expensive. Please do not take the synthetic D or DL forms of carnitine, as they can have negative side effects.

Carnitine comes in tablets or capsules, usually in 250 mg or 500 mg amounts. For fat burning and improved brain function I recommend 1,000 to 2,000 mg daily on an empty stomach, in divided doses. In other words, take 500 mg three or four times a day. As a maintenance and prevention supplement you can take 250-500 mg daily.

Vitamin C will greatly enhance your body's ability to use carnitine, so be sure you're getting at least 1,000 mg of vitamin C daily (which I recommend everyone take anyway) when you're taking carnitine. Carnitine's ability to improve alertness and attention can also cause insomnia in some people. If this happens to you, try taking the last supplement half an hour before dinner.

MEMORY AND ENERGY LOSS MAY BE A VITAMIN B12 DEFICIENCY

Many elderly people diagnosed with senility or Alzheimer's disease simply have a vitamin B12 deficiency. Vitamin B12, also called cyanocobalamin, plays a pivotal role in proper brain function.

The symptoms of B12 deficiency such as unsteady gait, fatigue and memory loss can begin showing up long before a blood test will show a deficiency. However, since the neurological damage done by a true B12 deficiency seems to be largely irreversible, it's not worth waiting around for it to show up that way. If you or a loved one is showing symptoms of a B12 deficiency, I highly recommend you find a health-care practitioner who will give 4-8 weeks of B12 injections to see if the symptoms improve. In the meantime, start using betaine hydrochloride and digestive enzyme supplements to improve digestion and absorption of nutrients. If a B12 deficiency is the cause of the symptoms, it will usually clear them up dramatically with a few weeks of injections.

Some people may need to continue getting regular B12 injections, and others may do fine maintaining with B12 supplements. It can be taken in supplement form as a nasal gel or sublingually, under the tongue. Vitamin B12 is not well absorbed when taken in pill form.

Magnesium is one of the magic minerals and it is essential to a high-energy lifestyle and brain power. The oxygen deficiency and muscle spasms caused by magnesium deficiency narrow the coronary arteries, interfering with heart function and impairing blood flow to the brain. A deficiency also makes the blood "sticky," which can contribute to having a stroke.

Nearly every important biological process in the body includes magnesium. Among its more important jobs are maintaining fluid and electrical balance in our cells, sending messages through the nerves, maintaining blood vessel strength, relaxing smooth muscles, keeping blood flowing smoothly, cholesterol balanced and the heart beating smoothly. It regulates how we absorb and use calcium and other minerals, and helps regulate how we use proteins and carbohydrates.

This magic mineral is also a key to energy production in the body, taking part in more than 300 enzyme reactions. The enzyme reactions regulate how the body uses nutrients and other substances such as hormones. For example, both vitamin B6, vitamin E and vitamin C need magnesium in order to work properly.

Magnesium can be depleted by stress, excessive alcohol, sugar, diabetes, kidney disease, chronic diarrhea, not enough protein in the diet, too much protein in the diet, and thyroid disorders. Drugs that can deplete magnesium include corticosteroids (Prednisone), loop and thiazide diuretics used to lower blood pressure (Diuril, Chlorothiazide, Oretic, Esidrix, Furosemide, Lasix, Bumex), aminoglycosides (antibiotics such as streptomycin, gentamicin and amikacin), and cisplatin (some chemotherapy drugs).

Magnesium by itself can cause diarrhea, so unless you are constipated, be sure to take it in a multivitamin, in combination with calcium, or in the form of magnesium glycinate or magnesium citrate. I recommend that you take 300-400 mg of magnesium daily as a supplement.

Coenzyme Q10 as an energy and memory booster is one of the best-kept secrets around. It is a vital enzyme, or catalyst to the production of energy in our cells. Without it, our cells simply won't work. Its chemical name is *ubiquinone*—it is ubiquitous, or everywhere, where there is life. Its levels in the human body are highest in the heart and liver. When we are ill or stressed, and as we age, our bodies are less able to produce CoQ10. Many older people who try CoQ10 report an almost immediate boost in their energy levels.

CoQ10 should come as a powder in a capsule, and be a deep yellow color. Also be sure that the product says "coenzyme Q10" or "CoQ10." Variations of it will not be as effective. The purity and quality of CoQ10 does vary, and since it's not a cheap supplement, it pays to get a high-quality brand. Most CoQ10 comes in 30 mg capsules. You can take one 30 mg capsule three times a day with meals, and up to 200 mg daily if your energy is low.

If you want to know more about CoQ10, get a paperback book called *The Miracle Nutrient: Coenzyme Q10*, by Emile G. Bliznakov, M.D. and Gerald L. Hunt (Bantam Books).

CHAPTER 6

Beating Depression Naturally

With very few exceptions, we all have cycles in our lives when we're down, cycles when we're up, and cycles when we're somewhere in between. It's quite normal to feel some level of depression before, during or after a major life change such as the death of someone close, illness or injury, birth, marriage, divorce, job change, or a move, for example. When we're very "high" or excited about something, we'll normally have a corresponding dip in our emotions. These emotional ups and downs are all part of being human, and most of us learn to cope with them pretty well by the time we're middle-aged. Debilitating depression that makes a person nonfunctional for weeks or months at a time is another story, and should be treated by a competent health care professional.

Minor depression can be a form of time-out for adults. Sometimes it's nature's way of giving us a rest, or perhaps we need to go within ourselves and be reflective. Maybe it's a message from the psyche telling us we need to reevaluate our lives. This reevaluation is most often an inner call to align ourselves with a sense of purpose, or mission in life—to go for what we *really* want, to reach for our dreams, even if they seem completely out of reach.

Unfortunately, thanks to a massive, multimillion-dollar public relations campaign on the part of the giant pharmaceutical companies who sell drugs such as Prozac, millions of people are suffering under the illusion that if they aren't feeling wonderful all the time, something must be wrong with them and they need to fix it by taking a pill. Never mind that the pills are expensive, addictive and have serious side effects!

Once you've had your time-out, or your grieving time, the first step toward healing depression is to get up out of bed, the armchair or off the couch, and *do* something, anything. Sweep the floor, go for a walk in the park, get a haircut, call a friend. Getting up and moving is one of the great cures for depression. Giving to others, forgiving others, and remembering what you're grateful for helps too. I realize this is easier said than done when you're *in* it, but go ahead and do it anyway!

If you're depressed to the point of being nonfunctional for weeks or months at a time, and haven't had any luck with conventional medicine, try to find a reputable alternative health-care professional. Very often, the skillful use of nutrition and supplements can help people with mild to moderate depression.

The most common physical causes of depression tend to be the same as those that cause a lack of energy: chronic stress, poor nutrition, lack of exercise. Some of us may be more genetically predisposed to have biochemical imbalances in the brain that contribute to depression.

AMINO ACIDS

Many alternative health-care practitioners have had great success treating depression with amino acids. Amino acids are the building blocks of protein and play a vital role in the production and regulation of brain chemicals. Most of the new "personality" drugs have much the same effects on brain chemistry as the amino acids tryptophan, L-tyrosine, and L-phenylalanine. These substances affect the brain's production of serotonin, a neurotransmitter that influences our moods. However, please try the simpler solutions such as nutrition and exercise first for treating depression—it's always preferable to begin with the most simple, down-to-earth solutions.

Although amino acids are safe, especially when compared to the prescription drugs, I strongly recommend that you not take more than the recommended dose unless so advised by a health-care professional, and monitor yourself carefully so you're tracking if and how they affect you. (Keeping a daily diary of how you're feeling works well.) The stimulating amino acids such as tyrosine and phenylalanine can cause irritability in some people.

If you have chronic, recurring depression, I would advise you to work with a health-care professional. Please do *not* take amino acids for depression if you are already taking a prescription drug for it, without consulting your physician.

If you, your physician or health-care professional want to know about amino acids in detail, I recommend the book *The Healing Nutrients Within* by Eric R. Braverman, M.D. and Carl C. Pfeiffer, M.D., Ph.D. (Keats Publishing, 1987). Your physician may want to check out some of the 120 pages of references cited. Very few prescription drugs have been so thoroughly tested.

Tryptophan

As I mentioned in the chapter on sleep, the amino acid tryptophan has, for all practical purposes, been banned by the FDA even though uncontaminated tryptophan is perfectly safe, and makes a wonderful antidepressant and sleep-aid. Ironically, tryptophan is still included in baby formulas and nutritional powders for senior citizens because it is an essential amino acid, but you can't get it by itself as a supplement in this country, even with a prescription. Tryptophan is often quite effective for treating depression, especially if there is an anxiety component to it, and if you have a reputable source outside the U.S., it may be worth trying.

L-tyrosine

L-tyrosine is fairly well established through research and the experience of hundreds of alternative health-care practitioners as a safe and effective remedy for depression. L-tyrosine is the precursor to some of our most important neurotransmitters, so it is an important part of our brain's nutrition. It is also a precursor to adrenalin, thyroid hormones and some types of estrogen. It has been shown to lower blood pressure, increase sex drive and suppress appetite. L-dopa, which is used to treat Parkinson's disease, is made from tyrosine.

Start with 500 mg three times a day with meals. If that doesn't work, try 1,000 mg. The most you should take without consulting a health professional is 1,500 mg. Although tyrosine is considered to be one of the safest amino acids, it can trigger a migraine headache in some people and shouldn't be used in conjunction with MAO inhibitors.

L-phenylalanine

L-phenylalanine is the precursor to tyrosine and has been used in numerous studies to successfully treat depression. Many supplement manufacturers will combine L-tyrosine and L-phenylalanine, but vitamin B6 should be added to this combination for better utilization.

This amino acid should be avoided by people who have PKU (phenylketonuria), a genetic defect in the body's ability to process and use phenylalanine. This defect can cause severe retardation. If it is caught early enough, retardation can be avoided with a phenylalanine-free diet. Some researchers believe that many children who are hyperactive or have learning disabilities are suffering from a mild form of PKU. Because there are a small number of women whose phenylalanine levels fluctuate when they are pregnant, this amino acid should be avoided if you are pregnant, just to be on the safe side.

The most common source of phenylalanine these days is the artificial sweetener aspartame (NutraSweet). Every time you use aspartame you get some phenylalanine and aspartic acid. However, I recommend you take phenylalanine in a supplement because we don't know enough about aspartic acid and its side effects, or what it does in combination with phenylalanine.

L-phenylalanine has been reported to raise blood pressure, so if you have high blood pressure please monitor it carefully or consult your physician. Phenylalanine gives some people headaches. A few studies suggest that L-phenylalanine may promote the growth of cancerous tumors, so if you have cancer this should not be your antidepressant of choice, and please avoid the aspartame! You can take up to 500 mg of phenylalanine three times a day.

THE B VITAMINS

The B vitamins play an essential role in our neurological health, and yet most adult Americans are deficient in them. Although each of the B vitamins plays some role in brain function, vitamin B12 is best known for its ability to combat depression. For years alternative-health professionals have given vitamin B12 shots as part of an overall treatment program for people who are extremely stressed out or depressed. Until recently this practice has been pooh-poohed, but now more and more M.D.s are jumping on the B12 bandwagon.

If you want to try B12 as an antidote for stress and/or depression, it's important to know that it's not well absorbed when you take it orally (by mouth), which is why it is given in the form of injections. However, there are B12 supplements you can buy at your local health food store that are sublingual (dissolve under the tongue) and intranasal (in the nose). You'll want to take about 1,000 mcg (1 mg) at least every other day for treating depression.

PRESCRIPTION DRUGS THAT CAN CAUSE DEPRESSION

One of the most common causes of depression is prescription drugs. Here is a list of some of the most common prescription drugs that can cause depression.

Amphetamines (including antihistamines)
Antibiotics
Anticonvulsants
Antidepressants (I kid you not!)
Barbiturates
High blood pressure drugs (beta-blockers, diuretics)

Hormones (estrogen, including Premarin, and
 synthetic progestins such as Provera)
Narcotics
Pain killers
Sleeping pills
Systemic corticosteroids (Prednisone, cortisone,
 etc.)
Tagamet and Zantac
Tranquilizers (Halcion, Librium, Restoril,
 Xanax, etc.)

CHAPTER 7

Working with Your Mind and Body to Beat Stress

While this is primarily a book about using nutrition to maintain an active lifestyle and handle stress effectively, exercise and the mind/body connection are such important factors in maintaining physical, mental and emotional balance that I felt it was necessary to include this chapter.

The word "stress" has its roots in the Latin for "narrow" or "tight." Have you ever felt the pressure of anxiety? Does your schedule keep getting tighter and tighter? Mental constriction is a familiar form of stress. We all know the physical expressions, too, revealed most obviously in the tightening of muscles. Bodily signs are easy to identify and offer an excellent opportunity to beat stress through relaxation. A physical approach, such as massage or exercise, will address adverse affects of stress in the body, including the build-up of toxic substances, sluggish circulation and shallow breathing. Any habit of physical activity also establishes a healthy substitute for time spent worrying. The best approach to relaxation, however, is a combination of mind and body work.

Working with the body redirects energy that has been channeled by emotional reactions that are stuck in a negative groove. Even mild resistance as you grit your teeth in heavy commuter traffic or do daily mundane chores after a long day manifests itself in tenseness somewhere in your body. Build in some form of physical exertion to your daily schedule and you will help undo the symptoms of stress.

The real key, however, is also to address the *causes* of stress. External pressures from career, relationships and money, for example, are often considered themselves as causes. The true origins of stress lie in our personal *reactions* to external factors. The mind has a tremendous capacity for retraining. People do lose the urge to smoke, drivers do stay calm in the face of road hogs, and even the boss has a lighter side to appreciate. Learn to focus your mind as well as your body and you will release the habitual thought patterns and responses which actually create stress.

EXERCISE

Exercise is a depression lifter. It stimulates the release of mood-enhancing chemicals in the brain and bloodstream. An aerobic workout is a much better immediate stress tonic than a cocktail or dose of caffeine. We instinctively recognize this when we take that walk round the block to "cool off." The pent-up energy is channeled in a healthy way. Establish a sensible exercise routine and you'll discover long-term benefits as moods lift and moderate.

Exercise also counters the draining effects of stress. Using physical energy actually trains the body to generate more. Get physically fit and your ability to meet stress increases. You will also build your resistance to illness, as moderate exercise has been shown to boost the immune system.

Stress leads to bad posture, poor breathing and harmful substances in the bloodstream. These physical signs are part of the tightening, clogging effects that come from feeling mentally strained. Exercise counters them all, and in a cyclical manner; improve one and the others tend to follow. Training the muscles of the body to overcome moderate resistance keeps them strong and toned. As tension relaxes, posture improves. Improved posture brings better breathing habits. Improve breathing and circulation becomes more efficient. Blood vessel networks expand, blood pressure improves and the heart grows stronger. Muscle tone increases with a better blood supply, and toxins are flushed out of the system, contributing to general well-being.

Exercise can help with specific forms of stress such as premenstrual syndrome (PMS) and insomnia. Improvements in digestion, metabolism and circulation that come with a regular physical workout result in better uptake of nutrients essential for trouble-free menstrual cycles and menopause, sleep and other bodily functions. The body's natural mood elevators and painkillers, called endorphins, circulate more freely with exercise. Research even shows exercise can improve short term memory.

The only downside for some people is the tendency to become exercise dependent, creating an inability to function normally without a workout "fix." If you find this happening, it's a sign that you need to work more with your mind. Relish your fitness, but expand your choice to include an Eastern approach such as yoga, chi gong or some form of meditation.

Your Exercise Choice

How do you include yet another activity in an already active life? Make it fun. Keep competition to a minimum, especially if it gets you worked up. Unless your exercise choice is pleasurable, you'll find it becomes another source of stress. Choose a sport to suit your character. Are you a sociable, team sports personality type or more of a loner, happy to squeeze in a daily workout? Are you an indoor, rowing machine sort or an outdoor jogger? Make your choice from the wide range of aerobic exercise to bring the cardiovascular benefits that will refresh and boost your system. Or take up a nonaerobic form such as yoga to condition your body and mind.

Walking, running, swimming, cycling, skating, racquetball, tennis, squash, jump-rope, stair climbing, rowing, and cross-country skiing are all excellent aerobic activities. Many of these adapt to intense, indoor aerobic exercise using equipment, which for some creates a more predictable and sustainable workout often better suited to city lifestyles. Don't ignore ordinary activities either, from vigorous house cleaning and raking the leaves to painting the house and pulling the weeds.

For standard exercise, aim at a minimum of twenty minutes a day. Build in a routine for five to six days a week, as this allows for necessary recovery time and lessens the tendency for addictive types to overdo it.

Take the time you need to select a suitable exercise and remember that about three months are needed to establish a new habit of any kind. Make sensible exercise a part of your routine and you automatically bring stress relief to your life.

BIOFEEDBACK

If you like hands-on technology, you'll enjoy biofeedback. Biofeedback is a form of body training that brings functions under conscious control that were previously subconscious. This type of training is ideal if you manifest stress in mainly physical ways. Biofeedback can be used to treat headaches, migraines, hypertension (high blood pressure), ulcers and digestive problems, for example. Biofeedback is also an aid in relaxation and meditation, as it can be applied to brain wave monitoring.

Our nervous system works on two levels—sympathetic and parasympathetic. The sympathetic system narrows blood vessels, raises blood pressure and speeds up heart rate. Under the parasympathetic system, heart rate is slowed, intestinal and gland activity increases, and sphincter (passage-closing) muscles relax. Biofeedback normally increases parasympathetic influence with the effect of slower heart rate for example.

In most biofeedback systems, your hand or some other part of your body will be hooked up to a machine sensitive to brain waves, body temperature or other body functions. It will beep or give you some other cue when you have achieved your goal: slower heart rate, lower body temperature or more relaxed brain waves, for example. The idea is to use a "soft" form of concentration to control the body, which can be surprisingly easy to achieve once you know how. The beeps are the feedback that let you know your focused thoughts and relaxation are having an effect.

There is a good reason for using skin temperature in biofeedback to beat stress reactions. Skin temperature increases when blood vessels are dilated, allowing blood to flow to the skin. Constriction of blood vessels is one effect of stress. This is an involuntary sympathetic nervous system response geared to conserve energy when it appears that the body is under threat. If you were asked to reverse this reaction and relax your body systems, it would be difficult to know where to start. Biofeedback shows you exactly what mindset and relaxation is needed to achieve control of this involuntary response.

Biofeedback tends to be very rewarding as you get better and better at producing the desired effects. Physical benefits can include the warming of hands and feet which have previously been permanent cold zones, relief from muscle tension, improved digestion, and lowered blood pressure and heart rate. Gaining practice at bringing the nervous system into balance is also practice for bringing the mind into focus in general.

Biofeedback Programs

It is not advisable to simply buy and use biofeedback equipment without formal training. Seek out an experienced therapist with an excellent reputation. Get recommendations if you can. Listings are found at hospitals and spas as well as in telephone directories. If your doctor refers you, you may find you are covered by your medical insurance. A good practitioner will offer a personalized program of about ten sessions, each about an hour long. A well-designed program will take you to the point where you are sure enough of the "bio" that you no longer need the feedback.

MEDITATION

Ever tried to "empty your mind" or obey a command *not* to think of a pink elephant? Meditation is not about banishing thoughts or blanking your mind. Meditation comes from the Latin "to think over." It means focused thinking. Some forms of meditation are used much like biofeedback. As with biofeedback, the physical results stem from a nervous system brought back into balance. Benefits are similar, including lowered heart rate and blood pressure, improved digestion and blood flow. Apparently Tibetan monks are even asked to demonstrate their meditative powers under extreme physical stress. The robes of the meditating monks are soaked with ice-cold water. The monks are said to have achieved the desired state when they have, by thought alone, increased their body temperature to the point where the robes are dried—not just once but six times in one long session!

The simplest meditation techniques are breathing exercises. A few minutes' concentration on deep, controlled breathing alone is a powerful tool, useful in everyday stressful situations. Cardiovascular benefits result as the body responds to the improved flow of oxygen. Calmness is felt as relaxation is induced.

Calmness and higher states of consciousness are often sought as aims of meditation. Many approaches are rooted in spiritual teachings from the East such as Zen Buddhism, although no religious beliefs are necessary to take up most forms of meditation. Some techniques require the repetition of a word or phrase. Others advise certain postures while some methods require only a relaxed sitting or lying position. Taking a course of instruction can make meditation a part of your social life, or a book can lead to a solo path. There are numerous books and classes which provide an introduction to a wide range of techniques. As your mind is your own, the choice is yours!

CHI GONG

Starting with either mind or body, stress is ultimately only fully addressed with a balanced approach to both. This seems to have been understood for centuries in the East. Many Eastern practices from martial arts and t'ai chi to acupuncture and meditation have been exported to the West. Part of the appeal of such techniques lies in the fact that they tend to involve the whole person, rather than isolating mind and emotion from physical expression. As such, Eastern disciplines make effective stress relievers. What is not well known is that chi gong lies at the root of such practices. The significant element in chi gong practice is becoming aware of and moving your energy, the very thing that is depleted or stretched to the breaking point with stress.

Also known as qigong, and chi kung, chi gong is the cultivation of energy. Chi, or ki, is the Chinese term for vital energy. Kung or gong means cultivation. By nurturing chi, the aim is to increase general health and well being. Many variations of its practice exist, but books such as *Chi Kung, Cultivating Personal Energy* by James Mac-

Ritchie (Element, Inc. 1993) are useful starting points. Seek out a reputable teacher for initial instruction when you are ready to integrate this ancient practice into your own life.

Simply explained, chi gong is a progressive series of calm, slow exercises, often in sets and involving concentration on breathing as well as movement. The aims for energy with chi gong are fourfold, aimed at it being balanced, free-flowing, of good quality and good volume. The exercises are meditative in that they ask for focus on specific chi points in the body, based on Oriental theories of anatomy and physiology as practiced, for example, in acupuncture.

We instinctively adopt chi gong postures as we naturally stretch and relax. Lying with our hands behind the head as people do all over the world, for example, directs energy to a point at the base of the skull, helping to relax vessels in the lower brain from where functions such as temperature and heart rate are regulated. As with meditation and ordinary exercise, you will get the most out of chi gong when you have regular practice. Benefits can include clearheadedness, body toning, a boost to the immune system, improved lymph circulation, as well as improved blood flow, blood pressure and heart rate.

SOURCES FOR NATURAL PROGESTERONE CREAM

Kenogen, P.O. Box 5764, Eugene, OR 97405, (503) 345-9855. This is progesterone in vitamin E oil, called Progest-E Complex.

Professional & Technical Services, Inc., 621 S.W. Alder, Suite 900, Portland, OR 97205-3627. (503) 226-1010, 1-800-888-6814. They sell Pro-Gest, the best known of the progesterone creams.

INDEX

acetaminophen, melatonin and, 25
acetylcholine, memory and, 52
aches, stress and, 2
Addison's disease, glycyrrhizin and, 14
adrenaline, 12–13
   balance of, 12–13
   fatigue and, 7
   hormones, depletion of, 5
aging
   DHEA and, 15–16, 33
   estrogen and, 9–12
   hormones and, 6
   melatonin and, 22–24
   men and, 16
   sleep and, 22
   supplements and, 30
AIDS
   DHEA and, 33
   EFAs and, 34
   minerals and, 33
   vitamin A and, 31
air pollution, 2
alcohol, 2
   sleep and, 10
   melatonin and, 25
allergies, 29, 39–45
   causes of, 39
   remedies, sleep and, 21
   steroid hormones and, 5
Alzheimer's disease, 28, 49, 52
amikacin, 57
amino acids, 61–64
   brain power and, 47
aminoglycosides, 57
amphetamines, depression and, 65
androgen, 15
animals, cruelty to, 9
anti-inflammation, EFAs and, 34
anticholinergic drugs, 52
anticonvulsants, depression and, 65
antidepressants, 3
   brain fog and, 50
   cancer, 64
   depression and, 65
   sleep and, 19–20, 26
antihistamines, depression and, 65
antiobiotics, depression and, 65

INDEX

antipsychotics, brain fog and, 50
anxiety
  herbs and, 3, 27–28
  nutrition and, 3
  St. John's Wort and, 27
  stress and, 1, 67–76
  tryptophan and, 26
appetite suppressants, sleep and, 21
arthritis, glutathione and, 35
Aspartame, 49, 64
aspirin, melatonin and, 25
asthma
  allergies and, 40
  polyunsaturated oils and, 34
  progestins and, 8
astralagus, allergies and, 41
Atarax, brain fog and, 50
autoimmune diseases, 29

B vitamins, 31–32
  brain power and, 47
  depression and, 64–65
  sleep and, 22–23
barbituates
  brain fog and, 50
  depression and, 65
behavior, steroid hormones and, 5
benzodiazephines, melatonin and, 25, 28
beta blockers
  brain fog and, 50
  depression and, 65
  melatonin and, 25

beta-carotene, vitamin A and, 30
biofeedback, 71–73
bioflavonoids, vitamin C and, 32
birth defects, folic acid and, 31
bleeding, progestins and, 8
bloating, estrogen and, 7–8
blood pressure drugs
  biofeedback and, 71–73
  depression and, 65
  ephedra and, 42
  glycyrrhizin and, 14
  salt and, 14
  steroid hormones and, 5
  stress and, 2
blood sugar
  brain power and, 47–49
  complex carbohydrates and, 37
bone growth, progesterone cream and, 10–11
brain power, 47–58
brain, cancer of the, 31
breast
  cancer, 10
  tender, estrogen and, 7–8
breathing, 67
  meditation and, 74
bromelain, quersetin and, 44
Bronkaid, sleep and, 21
Bumex, 57

caffeine, 2
  fatigue and, 12
  melatonin and, 25
  sleep and, 17, 20–21

calcium, 57
  sleep and, 22–23
calcium-channel blockers,
    melatonin and, 25
cancer
  antidepressants and, 64
  EFAs and, 34
  estrogen and, 7
  folic acid and, 31
  glutamine and, 53
  immune system and, 29, 33
  stress and, 2
carnitine, memory and, 53–54
cervix, cancer of the, 31
chamomile tea, sleep and, 21
chemotherapy, glutamine and, 35
chi gong, 36
  stress and, 75–76
Chlorothiazide, 57
cholesterol, hormones and, 6
chronic fatigue syndrome, 5
cigarette smoking, 2
circulation, exercise and, 69
cisplatin, 57
codeine, 14
coenzyme Q10, memory and, 58
coffee. See caffeine.
colds and flu
  allergies and, 40
  echinacea and, 36
  exercise and, 36
  medications, sleep and, 21
  melatonin and, 25

colitis, stress and, 2
colon, cancer of the, 31, 33
constipation, 37
corticosteroids, 57
  melatonin and, 25
cortisol, 5, 12
cortisone
  depression and, 66
  sleep and, 21
cysteine, 36

d-alpha tocopherol, 32
Dalmane, brain fog and, 50
dehydroepiandrosterone (DHEA), 5
  adrenal glands and, 15–16
  immune system and, 33
depression, 3, 59–66
  antidepressants and, 19–20
  estrogen and, 7–8
  herbs and, 3, 27–28
  nutrition and, 3
  St. John's Wort and, 27
  sleep and, 18
  stress and, 2
DHEA. *See* dehydroepiandrosterone.
diabetes
  glutathione and, 35
  magnesium and, 57
diarrhea
  magnesium and, 15
  minerals and, 33
  vitamin C and, 14
diet. *See* nutrition.
digestion
  biofeedback and, 71–73
  exercise and, 69

INDEX

diosgenin, 11–12, 16
disease, stress and, 1
diuretics, 57
  brain fog and, 50
  depression and, 65
  melatonin and, 25
Diuril, 57
drugs
  prescription, 2
  sleep and, 17

echinacea
  allergies and, 41
  immune system and, 36
eczema
  allergies and, 40
EFAs. *See* essential fatty acids
emotions
  control of, stress and, 2
  immune system and, 30
energy, 5–16, depression and, 60
environmental toxins, 50
enzymes, hormones and, 6
ephedrine
  allergies and, 41–43
  sleep and, 21
Esidrix, 57
esophagus, cancer of the, 31
essential fatty acids (EFAs), immune system and, 34
estrogen, 6
  brain fog and, 49
  depression and, 65
  fatigue and, 7
  synthetic, 7
exercise, 2

exercise (*cont.*)
  antidepressants and, 20
  brain power and, 47–49
  colds or flu and, 36
  depression and, 61
  lymphatic system and, 36
  menopause and, 10
  selection of, 70–71
  sleep and, 17
  stress and, 67–71

fatigue
  adrenal glands and, 12
  estrogen and, 7
  insomnia and, 20
  stress and, 1
fats, 2
fetal malformation, progestins and, 8
fiber, 36
flour, refined white, 37
flu. *See* colds.
folic acid
  immune system and, 31
  sleep and, 23
fructooligosaccharides (FOS), 32–33
furosemide, 57
  sleep and, 21

gamma-aminobutyric acid (GABA), 53
garlic, allergies and, 42
gentamicin, 57
ginkgo biloba, memory and, 51
ginseng tea, sleep and, 21
glucose
  tolerance, progestins and, 8

glucose (*cont.*)
  brain power and, 47–50
glutamate, 48
glutamic acid, 55
glutamine, immune system and, 34–35
glutathione, 35–36
grapeseed extract, the immune system and, 44

hair growth
  estrogen and, 7
  progestins and, 8
Halcion, depression and, 66
headaches
  biofeedback and, 71–73
  estrogen and, 7–8
healing
  post surgery, 34–35
  zinc and, 33–34
heart disease, 10
  ephedra and, 42
  estrogen and, 7
  glutathione and, 35
  St. John's Wort and, 27
  stress and, 2
herbs, 2
  anxiety and, 27
  depression and, 27–28
hives, allergies and, 40
homeopathic remedies, immune system and, 44
hormones, 5–16
  brain, 5
  depression and, 65
  female, linoleic acid and, 43
  replacement therapy 6
  steroid, 5
  synthetic, 6–8

hot flashes
  estrogen and, 10
  sleep and, 17
hydrocortisone, 13
hyperactivity, children and, 63
hypertension, biofeedback and, 71–73

ibuprofen, melatonin and, 25
immune system, 29–37
  balance test for, 11
infections, 29
inflammation
  glycyrrhizin and, 14
  steroid hormones and, 5
insomnia
  antidepressants and, 19–20
  St. John's Wort and, 27
insulin regulation, steroid hormones and, 5
irritability
  estrogen and, 7
  stress and, 2–3

Japan
  breast cancer in, 10
  hot flashes in, 10
jet lag, melatonin and, 24

kava, 27–28

l-dopa, 65
l-phenylalanine, 61, 63–64
l-tyrosine, 61–63
Lasix, 57
lecithin, 52–53
leg cramps, 23

INDEX

leukemia, DHEA and, 33
libido, estrogen and, 7
Librium, 28, 66
licorice root, adrenal glands and, 13–14
lifestyle
  antidepressants and, 19
  brain power and, 47
  energy and, 47
  estrogen and, 9
  heart disease and, 10
linoleic acid, 34
  43
liver damage, progestins and, 8
lovastatin, sleep and, 21
lungs
  cancer of the, 31
  polyunsaturated oils and, 34

ma huang, allergies and, 41–42
magnesium
  adrenal glands and, 14–15
  memory and, 56–58
  sleep and, 22–23
manganese, immune system and, 34
massage, stress and, 67
meditation
  adrenal function and, 12
  sleep and, 18
  stress and, 73–75
  the word, 74
melatonin, sleep and 22–25
memory loss, 48–50
menopause
  estrogen and, 7

menopause (*cont.*)
  hormones and, 6, 11
  sleep and, 17
  exercise and, 69
menstrual periods, hormones and, 6
mental alertness
  adrenal glands and, 12
  estrogen and, 7
  kava and, 28
metabolism, exercise and, 69
migraines
  biofeedback and, 71–73
  progestins and, 8
milk thistle, allergies and, 43
minerals
  hormones and, 6
  immune system and, 33
mint tea, sleep and, 21
miscarriage, progestins and, 8
monosodium glutamate (MSG), 48–39
moods, steroid hormones and, 5
Mormon tea, allergies and, 41–42
moving (changing residence), stress and, 1
MSG. *See* monosodium glutamate.
muscle weakness, adrenal glands and, 12
mushrooms
  allergies and, 41–42
  immune system and, 37

INDEX

n-acetyl cysteine, 36
narcotics, depression and, 66
Nembutal, brain fog and, 50
neurotransmiters, 5
niacin, memory and, 53
night sweats, sleep and, 17
NSAIDs (nonsteroidal anti-inflammatory drugs), sleep and, 25
Nutrasweet, 49, 64
nutrition
  adrenal function and, 12
  diet pills, melatonin and, 25
  estrogen and, 9
  heart disease and, 10
  men and, 16
  osteoporosis and, 10
  women and, 16

omega-3, immune system and, 34
Oretic, 57
osteoporosis
  estrogen and, 7, 10
  kava and, 27–28
  progesterone cream and, 10–11
oxygen, brain power and, 47–49

pain, stress and, 2
pain killers
  depression and, 66
  kava as, 27–28
  sleep and, 21
pantothenic acid
  adrenal glands and, 15

pantothenic acid (*cont.*)
  immune system and, 31
  memory and, 52
Parkinson's disease, 28, 52, 63
Paxil, 3
  sleep and, 19–20
PCOs, immune system and, 44
perfection, personal, 2
phenylalanine, 61
phenylketonuria (PKU), 63–64
phosphatidylcholine, 52–53
Ping Chuan Pill, 45
PMS, progesterone and, 8
polyunsaturated oils, 34
Prednisone, 13
  depression and, 57, 66
  melatonin and, 25
  sleep and, 21
pregnancies
  hormones and, 6
  folic acid and, 31
  vitamin A and, 31
Premarin, 7–9
  depression and, 65
premenstrual syndrome (PMB), 69
Prempro, 7
prescription drugs, brain and, 50–51
Primatene, sleep and, 21
proanthocyanidins. See PCOs.
Probiotics, immune system and, 32–33
progesterone, 6–7
  cream, 9–12, 76–77
  fatigue and, 7

INDEX

progesterone (*cont.*)
  menopause and, 8–9
  natural, 8–9
  synthetic, 7
progestins, 8, 10
  depression and, 65
propranolol, sleep and, 21
prostaglandins, 34
43
prostate problems, sleep and, 17
protein, osteoporosis and, 10
Provera, 7–8
  depression and, 65
Prozac, 3, 60
  brain fog and, 50
  sleep and, 19–20
  tryptophan and, 26
pseudoephedrine, sleep and, 21

quercetin, allergies and, 44

radiation, glutamine and, 35
rash, allergies and, 40
refined foods, brain power and, 47–49
reproductive organs, estrogen and, 7
rest
  adrenal function and, 12
  stress and, 37
Restoril, depression and, 66

salt, fatigue and, 14
saw palmentto, sleep and, 17
selenium, immune system and, 33
Serax, 28
sex characteristics, steroid hormones and, 5
sex drive, steroid hormones and, 5
silymarine, 43
sleep, 2, 17–28
  adrenal function and, 12
  brain fog and, 49
  depression and, 66
  exercise and, 69
  melatonin and, 22–25
  memory and, 51
  sleeping pills and, 22, 26
  stress and, 1
  tryptophan and, 26
soy products, menopause and, 10
spiritual balance, immune system and, 30
St. John's wort, 27
streptomycin, 57
stress 1–3, 67–77
  adrenal glands and, 12
  adrenaline and, 13
  depression and, 60
  fatigue and, 5
  professional therapy and, 18
  sleep and, 17–18
  the word, 67
  vitamin B6 and, 32
  women and, 32
stroke
  estrogen and, 7, 10
  progestins and, 8
  women and, 8
Sudafed, sleep and, 21

sugar, 2
  fatigue and, 12
suicidal behavior, 3
supplements, 2, 29–37
  adrenal glands and, 13–15
  aging and, 30
  sleep and, 22
synthroid, sleep and, 21
systemic corticosteroids, depression and, 66

Tagamet
  brain fog and, 50
  depression and, 66
teas, herbal, sleep and, 21
Tedral, sleep and, 21
testosterone, 6
  antidepressants and, 20
  fatigue and, 7
  synthetic, 7
theophylline, sleep and, 21
thyroid metabolism, steroid hormones and, 5
tranquilizers, memory and, 51
tryptophan, 26, 61–62
tumors, EFAs and, 34
tyrosine, 61

ulcers
  biofeedback and, 71–73
  glycyrrhizin and, 14
urinating, sleep and, 17

vaginal dryness, estrogen and, 10
Valium, 3, 28
  brain fog and, 50
  melatonin and, 25

vegetables
  immune system and, 37
  menopause and, 10
violent behavior, 3
viral diseases, 29
vitamin A, 30–31
  zinc and, 34
vitamin B12
  energy and, 56
  folic acid and, 31
  memory and, 56
  depression and, 64–65
vitamin B3, adrenal glands and, 15
vitamin B5, *See* pantothenic acid.
vitamin B6
  adrenal glands and, 15
  leg cramps and, 23
  immune system and, 32
  allergies and, 43
  magnesium and, 57
  L-phenylalanine and, 63
vitamin C
  adrenal glands and, 14
  immune system and, 32
  glutathione and, 35
  magnesium and, 57
  memory and, 55
vitamin E
  immune system and, 32
  glutathione and, 35
  magnesium and, 57
vitamins B. *See* B vitamins.

walking, stress and, 18
water, 2, 36, 47
  allergies and, 41
weight, body
  adrenal glands and, 12

INDEX

weight, body (*cont.*)
  brain power and, 47–48
  estrogen and, 7–8, 10
  stress and, 1
withdrawal behavior, 3
women, stress and, 32
  DHEA and, 33

Xanax
  depression and, 66
  melatonin and, 25

yoga, adrenal function and, 12

yogurt
  allergies and, 42
  immune system and, 37

Zantac
  brain fog and, 50
  depression and, 66
zinc
  immune system and, 33–34
  vitamin A and, 34
Zoloft, 3
  sleep and, 19–20

Dr. Earl Mindell's

What You Should Know About...
series
AVAILABLE NOW

Beautiful Hair, Skin and Nails
Better Nutrition for Athletes
Creating Your Personal Vitamin Plan
Fiber and Digestion
Herbs for Your Health
Homeopathic Remedies
Natural Health for Men
Natural Health for Women
Nutrition for Active Lifestyles
The Super Antioxidant Miracle
Trace Minerals
22 Ways to a Healthier Heart